OBESITY UNVEILED

How To Curb Your Appetite Shed Weight And Be Energetic

By

Mary J. Douglas

TABLE OF CONTENTS

INTRODUCTION

Weight loss is a goal for many people, although it is not the only way to improve your health. If you want to reduce your

weight, you must seek to do so through methods that will also promote your overall health. These habits include boosting your protein, fiber, water, and essential nutrients intake and eating enough to maintain your daily activity

with a modest shortfall to promote weight reduction. Eat well and eat right. Do not skip breakfast because it is very crucial for weight loss. Reducing calories involves establishing a calorie deficit by eating less than you burn each day. This method is how your body might shed weight over time. There are several methods you can limit your calories to encourage a healthy, balanced weight. If weight loss is your objective, then read on to learn how to trim calories healthily with backed up solutions.

Everyone overeats from time to time. Be gentle on yourself. It may help to understand why you eat and what occurs in your body when you eat or (overeat). Doing some activities and drinking water should help reduce the discomfort from overeating. While occasional overeating is fine, if you overeat more regularly, you may gain weight or develop chronic illnesses.

Individuals who are overweight or obese are at increased risk of several major diseases and disorders than people of healthy weight. These diseases consist of type 2 diabetes mellitus, chronic heart diseases, gallstones, etc. There are various probable contributors to obesity. The fact that the two main ones, diet and activity are ones you can influence is excellent news. A healthy lifestyle that puts exercise and food at its centre can also bring countless other health benefits. The more excessive your weight is, the more resistant your muscle and tissue cells become to your insulin hormone.

If you already are overweight or have obesity, these measures can also help you lose weight. Although it can be tough at times, it is truly a journey well worth pursuing.

CHAPTER 1

OBESITY AS AN EPIDEMIC

Obesity has been defined as a body mass index (BMI) greater than 30 kg/m2, with extreme obesity defined as a BMI larger than 40 kg/m2.

Obesity is connected with an increased incidence of several disorders, including diabetes, cardiovascular disease, and cancer. Consumption of fast food, trans fatty acids (TFAs), and fructose combined with growing portion sizes and decreased physical activity has been cited as a potential contributing cause of the obesity issue. The use of body mass index (BMI) alone is of low utility for predicting unfavourable cardiovascular outcomes, however, the efficacy of this measure may be strengthened when paired with waist circumference and other anthropometric parameters. Some public health programs have helped to identify and reduce some of the variables contributing to obesity.

The obesity epidemic will certainly impact practice for gastroenterologists since adjustments will be noticed in the incidence of obesity-related gastrointestinal illnesses, disease severity, and the pattern of comorbidities. The knowledge obtained with prior epidemiologic concerns such as smoking should allow concerned parties to expand needed health activities and raise the possibility of preventing future generations from enduring the repercussions of obesity. Obesity is fast becoming the largest cause of preventable deaths in the United States, with obesity-related fatalities estimated to shortly overtake deaths attributable to tobacco consumption. The rate of obesity has risen in the United States since 1960, with one-third of the adult population presently obese. Perhaps more worrying is the surge in overweight children. Many comorbid disorders have been related to obesity, including type 2 diabetes, hypertension, hypercholesterolemia, hypertriglyceridemia, and nonalcoholic fatty liver disease. As a result of these comorbidities, the medical expenditures directly associated with obesity are difficult to establish, but a conservative estimate would set the healthcare burden for obesity at around $150 billion per annum. The rapidly expanding population prevalence of obesity in recent decades has been attributed to an "obesogenic" environment, which allows quick access to high-calorie meals but limits possibilities for physical activity. The obesity pandemic can be regarded as a communal response to this environment. Obesity is a major public health problem because it raises the chance of acquiring diabetes, heart disease, stroke, and other serious disorders.

Any explanation of the obesity pandemic has to account for both heredity and the environment.

CHAPTER 2

OBESITY AND GENES

What exactly is the relationship between your weight and your environment and how much is influenced by your genes?

Children with obese parents have an 80% probability of being obese themselves, according to research on families and obesity. You could be tempted to believe that the genetic predisposition of the family plays the largest role in this, but studies have shown that only a little portion of this 80% chance is explained by the genetic relationship between weight and family history. Your family situation seems to be more important.

Not everyone develops obesity, even in an environment that promotes it. Indirect scientific evidence suggesting a large amount of the diversity in adult weight related to hereditary variables was available before the era of genomic research in studies of family members, twins, and adoptees. For instance, a significant study comparing the body mass index (BMI) of twins raised either together or apart discovered that hereditary characteristics had a greater impact than childhood environments.

Rare genetic variations have been linked to single-gene (monogenic) obesity so far, with at least nine genes being affected. There is typically no one genetic factor that causes obesity in an individual. More than 50 genes have been linked to obesity in studies, most with negligible effects. Several of these genes also have variations linked to monogenic obesity, a characteristic seen in numerous other prevalent diseases. The majority of obesity cases appear to be multifactorial, or the consequence of intricate interactions between numerous genes and environmental variables.In populations where the environment encourages inactivity and increased intake of high-calorie meals, obesity levels will escalate. However, not everyone who lives in these conditions will develop obesity, and not all obese persons will have the same body fat distribution or have the same health issues. The human populace's genetic changes happen too slowly to be the cause of the obesity pandemic. Nonetheless, the variance in responses across individuals to the same environment raises the possibility that genes are involved in the emergence of obesity.

How Do Genes Regulate The Balance Of Energy?

By responding to signals from adipose (fat) tissue, the pancreas, and the digestive system, the brain controls how much food is consumed. Hormones like leptin, insulin, and ghrelin, as well as other tiny molecules, carry these signals. These signals are coordinated by the brain with other inputs, and it then gives the body one of two instructions: either to consume more and expend less energy, or the reverse. The signals and reactions that regulate ingestion tendencies are based on genes, and slight adjustments to these genes' sequences can modify how active they are.

For survival, energy is essential. Instead of regulating weight increase, human energy management is designed to guard against weight loss. It was suggested that this observation could be explained by the "thrifty genotype" theory. That implies that places, where food is abundant all year round, are now challenging the same genes that enabled our ancestors to endure periodic famines.

Dynamics In Families And Weight

To help identify persons at high risk of obesity-related disorders like diabetes, cardiovascular diseases, and various types of cancer, healthcare professionals routinely collect family health histories. The influence of shared habitat and genes among close relatives can be seen in the family health history. Families have no control over their genes, but they may alter their surroundings to promote a balanced diet and regular exercise. These adjustments can enhance family members' health and the future generation's family health history.

CHAPTER 3

AN ELUCIDATION OF CALORIES

Energy is measured in calories. Nutritional calories are attributed to the energy that humans obtain from the foods and liquids they consume as well as the energy they expend when engaging in physical activities.

All food packaging contains information about nutrients and their calorie count. The main focal point of many weight loss plans is calorie restriction. The health of humans depends on calories and the secret is, getting the right daily quantity. Depending on their age, sex, size, and level of activity, each person needs a different amount of energy every day. Fast food accounts for more than 11% of daily calories consumed in the United States.

Foods containing lots of energy but few nutritional value are empty calories.

Although most people only think of calories in terms of food and beverages, anything that contains energy also contains calories. For example coal has a calorie content of 7,000,000 per kilogram (kg).

Two different kinds of calories exist, namely small and large calories.

- The amount of energy needed to increase the temperature of 1 gram (g) of water by 1 degree Celsius (o C) is known as a tiny calorie (cal).
- The quantity of energy needed to raise one kilogram (kg) of water by one degree Celsius is known as a big calorie (kcal). 1,000 calories make up one kcal.

It is usual to make use of the terms "big calorie" and "little calorie" interchangeably. This is deceptive. Large calories are used to describe the calorie contents on food labels. A 250-calorie chocolate bar has a caloric content of 250,000.

The average American needs 2,700 kcal per day for men and 2,200 kcal for women, according to the US government. Everybody's daily caloric requirements differ. Certain people have more vigorous lifestyles than others, and various people have distinct metabolisms that burn energy at different rates. The number of calories that should be consumed each day varies on many variables, including:

- General Health
- Physical activities
- Sex, weight, height, and body type

Diet And Calories

To survive, the human body needs calories. In the absence of energy, the body's cells would perish, the heart and lungs would cease beating, and the organs would be unable to perform the fundamental functions required for survival. People would most likely live healthy lives if they purely ate the necessary number of calories each day. Health issues will eventually result from eating too few or too many calories.

We can calculate the amount of potential energy a food has by counting its calories. Important factors include the source of the calories as well as the number of calories consumed. The calorie counts for three of the primary ingredients in the food are listed below:

- There is 4 kcal in 1 g of carbs.
- There is 4 kcal in 1 g of protein.

- There is 9 kcal per gram of fat

The body can use calories more efficiently if you eat a substantial breakfast. How well a person's body burns calories can be influenced by the time of day they consume. According to research, a substantial breakfast with about 700 kcal is best for promoting weight loss and reducing the risk of diabetes, heart disease, and high cholesterol.

A hearty breakfast may aid in maintaining a healthy weight. As important as what individuals eat is when they eat it.

- Filler calories

Energy-dense calories with scant nutritional value are known as empty calories. Food components that supply empty calories primarily come from added sugars and solid fats; they hardly ever contain dietary fiber, amino acids, antioxidants, dietary minerals, or vitamins.

- Soluble fats

Even though they are naturally present in many foods, they are frequently added both during industrial food processing and during the preparation of some dishes. An illustration of solid fat is butter.

- Added sugars

Sweeteners that are added to foods and beverages during industrial processing are known as added sugars. They contain lots of calories. The most popular added sugars in the US are sucrose and high-fructose corn syrup.

It is believed that added sugars and solid fats enhance the flavour of foods and beverages. Nonetheless, they significantly contribute to obesity and add a lot of calories.

- Alcohol

Alcohol may also add pointless calories to your diet. A typical serving of beer can increase a person's daily calorie consumption by 153 kcal.

If beer is not your preferred beverage, you can use a calorie counter to see how many calories drinking your preferred alcoholic beverages contribute to your diet.

The following foods and beverages contain the most empty calories:

- Additional sugars and solid fats
- Icy desserts, donuts, pastries, cookies, cakes
- Hot dogs, bacon, ribs, sausages, cheese, pizza
- Fruit juices, sports beverages, sodas, energy drinks

The leading single source of calories in the American diet is sugar-sweetened beverages, which also provide roughly half of the added sugars that consumers consume. The majority of Americans do not have room in their diets for a beverage that contains no sweetners at all. More than one sugar-sweetened beverage consumed each day raises the risk of high blood pressure, according to a recent study. It is preferable to stay away from them altogether and drink water, fat-free or milk with 1% fat, 100% fruit juice, and low-sodium vegetable juices instead. Fresh, healthy food and drinks can be included in the diet to prevent or significantly minimise the consumption of empty calories.

CHAPTER 4

THE CALORIE REDUCTION INACCURACY

For some people, reducing weight is not the ideal outcome, and being healthy is not the same as decreasing weight. Yet, 74% of adults in the United States are overweight or obese, which raises the risk of type 2 diabetes, several malignancies, cardiovascular disease, and other chronic health issues. If you want to know whether losing weight is a good aim for you, go to a healthcare professional.

Cutting calories results in a calorie deficit, which means that you are consuming fewer calories than you are expelling through your metabolism and daily activity. This calorie deficit helps you lose weight. Loss of tissue mass occurs when you eat fewer calories than you expend because your body cannot support all of its tissues. Larger part of the tissues you lose consists of muscle and fat mass.

As one pound of body weight equals 3,500 calories, many diet plans are centered on restricting your weekly calorie consumption by 3,500 calories or more to lose at least one pound of weight per week. The body is more complicated than a mathematical calculation, so weight reduction frequently does not proceed in this manner. It can progress more quickly or more slowly and is influenced by several things, including hormones and digestion.

Avoid Reducing Too Many Calories

As you reduce your caloric intake, your body will battle to maintain your weight. Although it may be annoying, your body's physiological safeguards against weight loss have developed to help people avoid starving and survive periods of famine. This is less useful for many people trying to lose weight in the modern environment.

By triggering these natural mechanisms early on in a weight-loss endeavour, cutting too many calories can be counterproductive. This involves changes in hormone levels, such as an increase in the hunger-inducing hormone ghrelin.

When you do not eat enough to support the movement, you can also find that you end up moving your body less since you have less energy and feel exhausted. When this occurs, you may wind up burning fewer calories throughout the day than you had been, which reduces or even eliminates your calorie deficit and slows or stops weight reduction.

Why It Is Not A Good Idea To Lose Weight Quickly And What To Do Instead

The 3,500-calorie calculation is a great beginning point even though it does not always accurately predict weight loss. The CDC advises losing 1 to 2 pounds each week in weight. A 500–1,000 calorie daily caloric deficit would be necessary to achieve this. Many people find this degree of a calorie reduction to be too excessive, and some experts advise never going below 1,400 calories per day. It is best to talk to a qualified dietitian or physician about your optimum calorie reduction goal. You can use a calorie calculator to estimate a calorie goal for weight loss that would be good for you, but bear in mind that this is merely a rough estimate and that your requirements might vary.

Get A Free Food Plan and Your Calorie Goal

Your metabolism has likely slowed as a result of hormonal adjustments if you have been restricting calories for a long period or have restricted them in the past only to gain weight. More calorie restriction might not be an effective technique for you in this situation. Your body may need more calories for a while, or you may need to rely on good nutrition and activity to speed up the healing process. Reducing calories does not always require you to weigh and measure your food on a scale or to count them. Although those methods can be successful, there are many other ways to lower your calorie intake.

How to Consume Fewer Calories

Cut back on portion sizes
Minimize calorie-rich beverages.
Change your diet
Take in plenty of fiber, protein, and water
Decrease your caloric intake during preparation.

- Cut back on portion sizes

A wise way to naturally create a calorie deficit is to reduce your regular meal portion sizes. It is recommended to start slowly and try to eliminate little portions of food gradually from each meal, modifying as necessary to notice results.

Using a smaller dinner plate is a simple approach to reducing your portion sizes. Naturally, eating from a smaller plate can result in consuming less food. Instead of using larger dinner plates, you might use a side or salad plate.

- Portion Size Calculation for Weight Loss

Using your hands as markers for the optimal portions in each meal is another approach to gauging portion proportions. Your hand makes it simple to estimate portions without a scale because it is easy and normally varies in size depending on your body size.

- How to Calculate Portion Sizes with Your Hand.

Fruits, grains and starches: Decide on a sum that is the size of your fist.

Vegetables: Choose only what your two hands can support.

Meat and substitutes: Choose a quantity that fits in your palm and is as thick as your pinky finger.
Fats: Choose a thumb's worth of fats.

- Limit Calorie-Dense Beverages

Drinks with a lot of calories might easily result in caloric excess. Particularly high-sugar beverages add calories and frequently do not offer any nourishment or a way to keep you feeling full. To promote healthy weight loss and maintenance, the USDA advises reducing foods and beverages with a lot of added sugars.

Instead of drinking your calories, eat them instead to avoid overconsumption. It is also unlikely that you would be able to offset the calorie intake from soda by exercising because drinking soft drinks is linked to weight gain whether or not you are physically active.

- .Skip the alcohol

For many people, cutting back on alcohol is a simple approach to losing weight. Alcohol has no nutritional value, so when you imbibe (drink) it, you are consuming empty calories. If you do order a drink, go for a 5-ounce (145 mL) glass of wine or a 12-ounce (355 mL) light beer (103 calories) (120 calories).

- Exchange foods.

Even though they are low in nutrients, you do not need to stop eating foods with a higher calorie count that you enjoy. The moderate use of higher-calorie foods can be a component of a healthy diet and happy lifestyle. Keeping these higher-calorie, less nutritious items to the occasional indulgence rather than a sizable portion of your regular diet is wise if you want your general eating pattern to encourage weight loss.

Using appropriate food substitutions that are pleasant and gratifying but lower in calories or higher in volume and nutrients, which encourages you to eat less than you otherwise would, is one approach to achieve this. To test some food swaps, here are some examples:

Replace some or all of the oil or butter in your baked products with applesauce.

In some savoury meals, low-sodium chicken stock can be used in place of butter, cream, or fat.

Substitute part or all of the spaghetti with zucchini or other vegetables.

Use of cauliflower as a rice substitute or thickener, or as a thickening agent in other recipes

Greek yoghourt, plain, non-fat, or low-fat, in place of sour cream

Use extra-lean ground beef or pig instead of cuts with more fat.

items made from whole grains rather than processed white products (bread, crackers, cereal, etc.)

- Get Your Fill of Fibre, Protein, and Water

Dietary components including fibre, protein, and water might help you fill up and be well satisfied for longer. They naturally limit your calorie consumption by filling you up and having an impact on how your digestive system works.

Your energy levels can be sustained and your blood sugar can be stabilised with a diet that includes a reasonable amount of protein and high-fibre carbohydrates. Consuming enough protein helps keep your muscle mass growth stable, which affects your metabolic rate. When trying to lose weight, it is important to maintain your muscle mass so that the majority of your weight loss comes from fat, which is not as metabolically active as muscle.

Compared to carbohydrates and lipids, protein is more satiating and satisfying. Naturally, you will want to eat less if you feel more satisfied and full. Moreover, protein takes longer to digest, which delays stomach emptying. Similarly to this, fibre slows down digestion and gives the food in your stomach and intestines more volume, causing you to feel fuller for longer.

Aim to meet or surpass the RDA for fibre while consuming more fibre. Adult men and women should each ingest 28 to 34 grams of fibre daily, and adult women should receive 22 to 28 grams.

- Choose Low-Calorie Preparation Techniques

Reduced calories throughout the day can naturally occur if you choose lower-calorie meal preparation techniques. There are additional techniques to reduce calories that can be utilised independently or in conjunction with healthy lower-calorie food changes like those already discussed.

Making your meals at home is the best strategy to reduce your calorie intake when it comes to food preparation. Meals from restaurants and fast food chains typically have greater calorie counts than meals made at home since you have more control over the components. Additional low-calorie preparation techniques include steaming, grilling, sautéing, baking in place of frying, and so on. You can cut back on the amount of oil needed for sautéing or cooking by using non-stick cookware. Avoid oil-frying your food to significantly reduce the number of calories you consume. Try using an air fryer if you like fried foods.

CHAPTER 5

THE BEHAVIOUR OF BINGE EATING

Overeating and eating past fullness are rather frequent behaviours. At parties, family reunions, and special occasions, we overindulge. Yet, overeating can also lead to obesity and the emergence of eating disorders.

Overeating is extremely prevalent and biological. Cortisol production in your body is increased when you are under stress. High cortisol signals the need to locate food among other things as part of the fight-or-flight response. You might start to crave foods high in salt, sugar, or fat. Several forces are also at work in this situation. Overeating can be influenced by how quickly you eat, what you eat when you eat, and what you do while you eat.

Periodic overeating can lead to indigestion and stomach pain, affect how your body controls hunger, and result in weight gain.

Significance And Causes

Signs of overeating
If you eat too much, you could have acid reflux, bloating, gas, heartburn, nausea, and stomach ache. You will also feel drained and slow. A few hours later, the discomfort from the overeating should start to subside. Exercise and drinking plenty of water could hasten your recovery.
In addition to overeating, there may be additional causes for similar symptoms. These symptoms could not be caused by overeating if they persist for more than a day. A healthcare physician should be contacted if they worsen or persist for a week

How Can You Tell When You Have Eaten Too Much?

Usually, your body uses hormonal signals to control hunger. When you have not eaten in a while, your ghrelin hormone levels increase, making you feel hungry. The leptin hormone alerts you to fullness after eating. These signals are suppressed by overeating and this throws off the hormones that control our hunger, increasing the likelihood that we may eat for pleasure rather than for hunger. Around 20 minutes after you finish eating, you might not realise you overate. Then, later you can feel fatigue or stomach discomfort.

What Triggers Binge Eating

Overeating can have a variety of causes, some of which are connected to the foods themselves and others to the context or timing of our meals. Overeating can result from various factors, such as: eating out of emotion. When you are under stress, unhappy, exhausted, bored, or depressed, you are more prone to eat. Endorphins are feel-good hormones that are released by eating. For this reason, a lot of people enjoy eating. We can do it if we are feeling stressed out or exhausted. We are more inclined to overeat when we eat because it makes us feel good rather not necessarily because we are hungry. Overeating is prevalent with foods like French fries, pizza, chocolate, and ice cream.

- Processed meals

You are encouraged to eat for enjoyment and to keep eating even when you are not hungry by processing and adding flavours.

- Time

In the evenings is when you are more likely to eat for pleasure rather than solely to get the energy your body requires, overeating is prevalent.

- Social circumstances

Humans frequently congregate around food - during celebrations, and sporting events, and to connect with family and friends. When you are in a social setting, you can be more easily distracted, uneasy, or under pressure to eat something even if you are no longer hungry while everyone else is eating. You tend to consume greater servings than necessary.

- Medications

You may become less aware of when you are full if you take certain drugs. If you start overeating following a drug change, consult your doctor.

- Ailments

Premenstrual syndrome, atypical depression, anxiety, Prader-Willi syndrome (PWS), and Kleine-Levin syndrome are a few medical illnesses that might lead to overeating

Control And Treatment

What should I do if I have eaten too much?

Feeling guilty or blaming yourself will not make you feel better if you overeat. Keep in mind that overeating is typical. It is crucial to be polite to yourself while your digestive system is working because you can feel bad for a few hours. You can take certain actions to aid your body in digesting your meal and assist you to get back on track. For instance:

- Go on a walk. Regulating your blood sugar and reducing gas are also benefits of modest exercise.
- Remain hydrated. More water will be required by your digestive system to process the additional weight.
- Teas made from herbs, such as peppermint, chamomile, and ginger, might improve digestion and lessen flatulence.
- Heartburn or indigestion may be relieved by taking an over-the-counter antacid.

Antacid side effects and complications

Constipation.

Diarrhoea.
The colour of your excrement changes.
Abdominal pain.

Even though it is common to occasionally overeat, doing so might alter how your body manages hunger and cause unintended weight gain. We frequently overeat because it makes us feel wonderful. Doing extra activities that make you feel good other than eating may therefore be helpful.

- Adopt good self-care habits: Do some exercise, get enough sleep (but not too much), and use social media sparingly.
- Use alcohol in moderation. When we are drinking, we eat more. Reducing spending might be beneficial.
- Eat less salty meals because it may make you crave sweets more.
- Vegetables, which provide more fibre and will make you eat more slowly, should take up the majority of your plate.
- Organise your tension. Hunger and fullness hormones can be suppressed by stress hormones.

- Consume gradually. If you take your time, you might feel full before your dish is completely finished
- Mindfully eat. Understand your eating triggers and purposes.
- Exercise frequently. An alternate way to get endorphins is through exercise.

A few times a year of binge eating should not result in long-term weight increase. However, it will if overeating develops into a pattern. Be kind to yourself if you start to feel uncomfortable after eating too much. Drink some water and engage in some modest exercise. Do not substantially cut back on calories the following day either. Eat when you are hungry and do so consciously.

Why Can Eating Too Much Make You Feel Exhausted?

When you eat too much, your body has to work harder and transfer blood to your active digestive system instead of other organs. This could make you feel drained or lethargic. The meals we tend to overeat also have a greater carbohydrate content, which can lead to a sugar rush and a subsequent sugar crash. Discussing your symptoms and eating habits with a healthcare professional may be beneficial if you find yourself overeating more frequently than once per week for a few months.

CHAPTER 6

OBESITY AND POVERTY

According to numerous news sources and government organizations, the United States is currently experiencing an "obesity pandemic." For good reasons, public health professionals and researchers are particularly worried about childhood and teenage obesity. Obesity among children has nearly tripled during the last three decades. While obesity is a problem for all American populations, the particular vulnerability of the most underprivileged communities is frequently overlooked. Particularly among Americans with the lowest levels of education and the highest rates of poverty, obesity is rife. It is crucial to comprehend why and how poverty exacerbates the growth in childhood obesity given the growing economic insecurity that many people in our country face today. We cannot successfully devise solutions to lower this significant health risk to already vulnerable people unless we are aware of the underlying reasons at play.

Why Poor People Have a Higher Obesity Risk

All people in America can choose to reduce their risk of obesity and related health issues by eating healthfully and exercising regularly. Of course, the family and community circumstances in which children and adolescents live have a significant impact on the decisions they make. Poor living conditions are important, especially for young people because they make it more difficult for them to engage in healthy habits.

Since they typically have to wait until the end of the month for their next check or Food Stamp allocation, low-income families frequently have to stretch their food budgets and selection. This results in unhealthy behaviour in several ways:

- Because they are less expensive and less perishable than fresh produce, lean meats, and fish, families prefer high-fat, calorie-dense foods like sweets, cereals, potatoes, and processed meats.
- Poor families frequently reside in underdeveloped areas where it is challenging to get wholesome nutrition. Little grocery stores and fast food restaurants that serve cheap, high-fat foods are more prevalent in disadvantaged neighborhoods than in big supermarkets. People frequently turn to high-fat, sugary foods to help them cope with economic uncertainty, which includes having difficulties paying their bills or rent.

- Poor people's options for regular physical activity may also be limited because they typically lack the resources to pay for organized after-school activities for their children and because schools in deprived areas are less likely to offer sports or physical activity programs than schools in wealthier areas.

- Poor parents, particularly single mothers, may find it difficult to finance extracurricular activities for their kids due to rigid work schedules, a lack of transportation, or unmet child care demands. That is frequently all that stressed-out, underprivileged parents can do to leave their children in front of the television.

- There are frequently no parks, playgrounds, trails, or free public gyms in many impoverished neighborhoods. There may be no adjacent indoor spaces for play or exercise, and neighborhoods may be rife with violence. In an ironic twist, parental efforts to keep their children safe and indoors may enhance the encouragement of sedentary activities like watching TV and playing video games.

Youthful Obesity's Long-Term Negative Effects

Adolescents from poor homes and communities have a higher likelihood of becoming fat as adults than those from wealthier backgrounds. Moreover, obesity in young adults is typically not transient. That is akin to receiving a life sentence of socioeconomic deprivation and poor health.

- Obese young adults are at significant risk for developing chronic illnesses like heart disease, depression, and specific malignancies.
- Young adulthood obesity is connected to lower levels of income, unemployment, and educational attainment.

Obesity needs to be avoided or reversed in underprivileged children since it has long-lasting and repeated negative effects.

What to do:

We have to think about the problems in more than simply individual terms if we want to effectively prevent and reverse obesity among especially vulnerable impoverished individuals. We must seek for approaches to start enhancing the social and natural surroundings in which low-income individuals live. Neighborhood and community institutions can benefit from interventions.

In order to connect neighbors and engage in safe, well-organized activities that promote both physical and mental health, new community resources are also required.

Due to the amount of time children spend there and their importance as respected local institutions, schools, and Head Start programs can also be important participants. According to research, the prevention of childhood and adolescent obesity can be greatly aided by including physical activity and a healthy diet in school and preschool programs.

CHAPTER 7

RELATIONSHIP BETWEEN OBESITY AND CANCER

If you are obese or highly overweight, your body has more fat than other tissues, like muscles and bones. You run a higher risk of developing some cancers and of having cancer recur after treatment if you carry too much additional weight.

It is crucial to discuss your weight with your doctor, but for some people, this can be challenging. Some people experience embarrassment because of their weight. Even prejudice against some persons because of their weight has occurred. Changing your habits, such as what and how much you eat and how much you exercise, can often feel overwhelming. But, even modest, easy changes can have a significant effect on your health.

It is critical to comprehend what experts in the field of cancer risk mean. Not everyone who develops cancer will also have risk factors, such as being overweight or obese. Understanding your cancer risk can help you make healthier decisions and help you be aware of the warning signs and symptoms.

The relationship between body weight and cancer risk is still being researched. There are various factors that weight might have on your risk of developing cancer. They consist of:

- Your levels of the hormones, insulin and insulin growth factor increase as you gain weight. A surplus of this hormone may contribute to the growth of some malignancies.
- Estrogen is also produced in greater amounts by fat tissue. Certain malignancies, like breast cancer, might spread more quickly due to estrogen.
- Obese individuals are more likely to experience chronic, low-level inflammation, which is associated with a higher risk of developing cancer.

The way your body controls the growth of cancer cells is impacted by fat cells.

Your lifetime weight fluctuations may also impact your risk of developing cancer. According to studies, the following variables can influence your risk:

- Greater birth weight than the majority of newborns
- Weight gain in adulthood
- Repeatedly losing weight and gaining it back

Your chance of developing cancer is decreased by eating a balanced diet, maintaining a healthy weight, and engaging in regular exercise. Making these healthy decisions can help reduce your risk of cancer recurrence if you have already had cancer before.

Being overweight or obese has been linked to the following cancers:
- Mammary cancer
- Ovarian cancer
- Prostate cancer
- Cancer of the pancreas
- Pancreatic cancer

- Thyrotoxic cancer
- Intestinal cancer
- Throat and head cancer
- Stomach cancer

Your "body mass index," or BMI, is a calculation that determines whether you are overweight or obese. It is determined by your height and weight. Depending on your race and physical characteristics, your BMI categorization and measurements may change. Although BMI is frequently used in studies to better understand how obesity and cancer are associated, it is not a reliable indicator of future health. Discuss the implications of your BMI for your risk of developing cancer with your medical team.

A standard BMI starts from 18.5 to 24.9. A BMI of 25 to 29.5 is regarded as overweight. A BMI of 30 or more is termed as obesity.

Your waist measurement is a different measurement you can take. According to research, those with greater waist measurements are more likely to develop specific ailments, such as cancer and heart disease. For men, a healthy waist circumference is under 40 inches (101.6 cm), and for women, it is under 35 inches (88.9 cm).

Keeping Your Weight Constant

You should take measures to maintain your weight if you are content with it and your medical team agrees, and you do not desire to lose or gain weight. Here are a few pieces of bits of advice:

- Consume a lot of fruits, veggies, lean proteins, and entire grains.

- Consume foods that fill you up, including fish, almonds, and healthy fats like olive oil and nuts.

- Steer clear of packaged foods with lots of artificial ingredients, white bread, cookies, and other highly processed foods.

- Avoid sugary beverages including soda, fruit juice, and other high-sugar beverages. Examine the sugar and calorie content of any alcoholic beverages and your coffee.

- Make it a point to get in 30 to 60 minutes of exercise most days of the week. Moderate or vigorous exercise is both acceptable. Go for a run, or a brisk stroll, or enrol in a fitness class. Do what you can if you can not obtain 30 to 60 minutes. Your risk of cancer is reduced even by a few extra minutes every day.

Find out how many calories you should consume each day by asking your healthcare professional. Keep to or as near to, your daily allowance. If you have been diagnosed with cancer, you should also discuss any worries you may have in advance with your cancer care team regarding modifications to your food or exercise routine as a result of your diagnosis or treatment.

Lowering Cancer Risk If You Are Obese Or Overweight

The greatest approaches to enhance your health if you are overweight or obese are to eat better and move more. The chances of developing cancer can be decreased by losing as little as 5% to 10% of your overall body weight. Although it might seem insignificant, research demonstrates that it can have a positive impact on your health. Eating a more balanced diet and staying active regularly can help lessen your chance of developing cancer, even if losing weight is difficult for you.

The following actions will assist you in choosing healthier options:

- Make minor adjustments to your diet and exercise regimen. Members of your healthcare team who can offer assistance if you struggle with eating less and moving more and assist you in making adjustments include a qualified dietitian, an exercise specialist, a psychologist, or a physician who focuses on weight loss.

- Get assistance. When attempting to modify one's lifestyle, it is critical to feel supported. Meetings with a dietician or weight loss expert are typically included in weight loss programs. They can assist you in making better choices and sustaining them over time. Ask for help from your relatives as you discuss the adjustments you wish to make. If the people you live with also make changes, it will be much simpler for you to do so.

- Medication. If diet and exercise are ineffective and your obesity is contributing to other serious health conditions, some medical professionals may advise taking medication.

- Surgery to lose weight. Weight loss surgery can be an option for you if you have a serious health condition linked to obesity, such as diabetes or heart disease. Bariatric surgery, often known as weight loss surgery, involves having your stomach reduced in size. Several types of weight loss surgery exist. Typically, this is only taken into account for persons who have a BMI of 40 or higher or 35 or higher with a major medical condition.

Working together with your medical team will help you lose weight and make healthy improvements. It might be challenging to maintain a healthy weight after experiencing rapid weight loss. Yo-yo dieting, often known as a cycle of losing and gaining weight, has been associated with a higher risk of developing cancer. Diets that do not provide you with all the necessary nutrients, such as crash diets, might be risky. Also, if you have ever struggled with an eating disorder, you should always consult your doctor before starting any new exercise or food regimen.

Questions To Put To Your Medical Team

For those wishing to reduce their risk of cancer in general:

- Do I have an increased chance of getting cancer because of my body weight?
- Will shedding pounds enhance my general health? Will it lessen my risk of developing cancer?
- What amount of weight should I shed?
- What services and remedies are offered to assist me in making dietary and exercise changes?
- Can you suggest someone assist me with a weight loss plan?
- Where can I obtain details about a healthy diet?

- What sources are there for information on exercise?

Survivors Of Cancer:

What advantages do changing my way of life have for my health?
- Would shedding pounds impact my chance of a cancer recurrence?
- Are there any workouts I should stay away from because of the illness or how it is being treated?
- Is there a specialist I may consult regarding my nutrition and exercise regimen, such as an oncology dietician or another professional?

CHAPTER 8

RELATIONSHIP BETWEEN INSULIN RESISTANCE, TYPE 2 DIABETES, AND OBESITY

One initiating factor for diabetes linked to insulin resistance is obesity. Adipose tissue in obese people releases increased levels of non-esterified fatty acids, glycerol, hormones, and pro-inflammatory cytokines that may contribute to the emergence of insulin resistance. Insulin resistance is also influenced by endoplasmic reticulum stress, adipose tissue hypoxia, oxidative stress, lipodystrophy, and genetic predisposition.

Type 2 diabetes mellitus is preceded by insulin resistance, which is also a contributing factor in the so-called metabolic syndrome. Insulin resistance can impact people with type 1 diabetes even though it is a feature of prediabetes and type 2 diabetes.

Knowing insulin resistance?

Individuals who have insulin resistance, sometimes referred to as decreased insulin sensitivity, have developed a tolerance to the hormone, which reduces its potency. More insulin is consequently required to convince fat and muscle cells to absorb glucose and the liver to keep storing it.

It is still unclear as to why a person does not react to insulin as intended. However, there are methods to increase the body's receptivity to insulin, which can assist people with type 1 diabetes control their blood sugar levels or prevent or delay the onset of type 2 diabetes (blood sugar).

The pancreas releases more of the hormone in response to the body's insulin resistance to keep cells active and blood glucose levels under control. This explains why individuals with type 2 diabetes frequently have high amounts of circulating insulin. Although the pancreas may produce more insulin, insulin resistance alone will not initially cause any symptoms. Yet, over time, insulin resistance deteriorates and the pancreatic beta cells that produce insulin may deteriorate. The pancreas eventually runs out of insulin to get past the cells' resistance. Higher blood glucose levels are the end effect, which can lead to type 2 diabetes or prediabetes.

The effects of insulin resistance are expected to extend beyond diabetes because insulin has several functions in the body other than control blood glucose levels. For instance, several studies have revealed a link between heart disease and insulin resistance, which is unrelated to diabetes.

Why Does Insulin Resistance Occur?

A risk factor for the development of insulin resistance is obesity. Increasing production of pro-inflammatory cytokines has been linked to increased adipose tissue, which, together with fatty acids, appears to be the cause of the emergence of insulin resistance. As a result, the expansibility or capacity of adipose tissue to store lipids, which varies depending on the individual, also appears to play a significant role in the development of insulin resistance because, if this capacity were to be exceeded, lipids would leak out into other tissues where they might disrupt insulin signalling.

The causes of insulin resistance are starting to become more clear to researchers. To begin with, it has been discovered that several genes influence a person's propensity to develop the ailment. Insulin resistance is also more common in elderly individuals. Lifestyle might also be a factor.

Insulin resistance testing is typically not done by doctors as part of routine diabetes therapy. However, when conducting clinical research, researchers may focus explicitly on indicators of insulin resistance, frequently to examine new therapies for either type 2 diabetes or insulin resistance. To prevent levels from falling too low, they often give a person a lot of insulin while also supplying glucose to the blood. The stronger the insulin resistance, the less glucose is required to maintain normal blood glucose levels.

Ways It Affects Your Health

The degree of insulin resistance varies. Since more medicine is required to get enough insulin into the body to attain goal blood glucose levels, the more insulin resistant a type 2 diabetic is, the more difficult it will be to treat their diabetes.

Type 1 diabetics who are insulin resistant will require higher insulin doses to maintain blood glucose control than those who are more insulin sensitive. Resistance to insulin is not a cause of type 1 diabetes. Like persons with type 2, those with type 1 may have a genetic propensity to develop insulin resistance or may do so as a result of being overweight. According to certain studies, type 1 diabetes patients' insulin resistance may contribute to cardiovascular disease and other problems.

The prevalence of type 2 diabetes mellitus (T2DM) is rising, and there are no indicators that this trend is slowing down due to global obesity. Although the apparent connections between obesity and type 2 diabetes mellitus, actual mechanisms are complex because some obese individuals seem to be somehow protected from acquiring type 2 diabetes mellitus. The metabolic syndrome, which includes obesity, type 2 diabetes mellitus, hypertension, and dyslipidemia, causes millions of individuals each year to die suddenly from cardiovascular disease. In addition to having a significant negative impact on quality of life, long-term microvascular complications from type 2 diabetes mellitus and the numerous comorbidities associated with obesity (psychological, musculoskeletal, respiratory, and reproductive) also place a tremendous financial burden on international health organizations. Diabesity is a concept that has been coined to describe the interdependence between diabetes and obesity. Chronic overconsumption of foods that are high in calories, lifestyle choices, genetic composition, and environment all play significant roles in the function or dysfunction of adipose tissue. Impaired fat metabolism along with glucotoxicity is a feature of type 2 diabetes mellitus Overeating meals that are high in energy leads to excessive fat deposition and increased insulin resistance. Fatty liver is caused by the delivery of free fatty acids (FFAs) to the liver through the portal vein. A viscous loop of fat destruction, inflammation, deteriorating insulin resistance, and beta cell insulin production, and eventually the evidence of type 2 diabetes mellitus rising is caused by FFAs spilling into the systemic circulation and causing lipotoxicity of organs like the pancreas, heart, and muscles. Visceral fat level is a reliable indicator of insulin resistance, but adipokines like adiponectin guard against the development of type 2 diabetes (T2DM) brought on by obesity. The development of new management and prevention methods for T2DM in the context of obesity will be made possible by further research into the precise mechanisms of lipotoxicity in the development of T2DM.

Correlations between obesity and T2DM

Due to its rising prevalence and a cluster of disorders, it is connected with that lower life expectancy and quality of life, obesity has become a serious problem on a global scale. Obesity is the abnormal accumulation of fat in the adipose tissue brought on by prolonged overeating, a lack of exercise, inherited factors, or both. Type 2 diabetes, heart disease, cancer, and early mortality are all risks of obesity. According to the most recent World Health Organization (WHO) estimates, the global rate of obesity has nearly doubled since 1990, and T2DM is also on the rise. Almost 1.1 billion individuals are thought to be overweight, with 320 million of them being considered obese. Higher BMI (body mass index) is thought to be a contributing factor in more than 2.5 million deaths annually; by 2030, this number is projected to double. Worldwide, there are roughly 300 million adult obese people.

T2DM is a diverse ailment that is most frequently characterized by insulin resistance, a condition of diminished insulin-mediated glucose uptake when pancreatic beta cells are unable to make and provide enough insulin to meet the body's needs. The beta cells are not irreversibly harmed after 2-3 years of T2DM, but if the energy overload continues for years, the beta cells become permanently impaired, necessitating the use of insulin to regulate blood sugar levels.

Since 80% of diabetics are obese, obesity and diabetes are strongly related to one another. With T2DM, obesity is a frequent finding. Peripheral tissues, such as muscle and fat cells, are less sensitive to the effects of insulin in obese people (insulin resistance). When such obese patients lose weight, their diabetes condition improves. Obesity raises the danger of T2DM, heart disease, cancer, and early demise. Lipoprotein lipase, which plays a crucial role in the metabolism of both triglyceride-rich particles and high-density lipoproteins, is a pharmacological component that contributes to obesity and diabetes (HDL). HDL and triglyceride levels in serum are determined by lipoprotein lipase.

It is commonly understood that people who are overweight or obese are more likely to develop type 2 diabetes, especially if they have extra weight around their stomachs (abdomen). Abdominal obesity triggers the release of "pro-inflammatory" chemicals from fat cells, which can reduce the body's sensitivity to the insulin it generates by interfering with the insulin-responsive cells' ability to operate. Insulin resistance, a significant risk factor for type 2 diabetes, is what this is. Obesity that is very perilous and is portrayed by excess abdominal fat (i.e., a big waistline) is referred to as central or abdominal obesity.

The location of fat accumulation and the degree of obesity both affect the impact of obesity on the risk of type 2 diabetes. Although underlying processes are unclear, increasing upper body fat, especially visceral adiposity, as seen in increased abdominal girth or waist-to-hip ratio, is linked to metabolic syndrome, type 2 diabetes, and cardiovascular disease

More research is needed to determine, for instance, if subcutaneous fat is merely a more neutral storage position or does not have the pathogenic implications of visceral fat. Despite variations in body fat distribution, the new data point to the possibility that various subtypes of adipose tissue may differ functionally and have diverse effects on glucose homeostasis. Brown fat cells, which play a function in thermogenesis and may have an impact on energy expenditure and obesity susceptibility in adult humans, are scarce and vary in quantity [15]. Investigation into the pathogenesis and problems of obesity must prioritize a better understanding of the operation of various fat cell types and depots, as well as their roles in maintaining metabolic homeostasis. Similar to other tissues, adipose tissue is made up of a variety of cell types. Adipose tissue immune cells are likely involved in systemic metabolic processes as well. It will be crucial to take into account if other adipocyte subtypes or other cell types can be discovered as the research of adipose biology advances to improve our comprehension of the consequences of obesity and develop fresh approaches to prevention.

Obesity has been associated with insulin resistance and has been linked to T2DM through at least three different mechanisms:

Lower levels of adiponectin and increased synthesis of adipokines/cytokines that promote insulin resistance, such as tumour necrosis factor-a, resistin, and retinol-binding protein ectopic fat accumulation and dysmetabolic consequences, especially in the liver and possibly in skeletal muscle; and decreased mitochondrial bulk function, which indicate mitochondrial malfunction One of the many significant underlying abnormalities connecting obesity to diabetes may be mitochondrial dysfunction, which impairs b-cell activity and lowers insulin sensitivity.

Obesity and T2DM have a significant impact on premature mortality, quality of life, associated chronic microvascular problems (in the case of T2DM), obesity-associated comorbidities, and the global healthcare sector, whether they exist alone or together as "diabesity." It is crucial to have a better knowledge of the therapeutic and causal interactions between these two disorders. Effectively combating the escalating global obesity epidemic will require a multifaceted strategy that targets both adults and children, as well as changes to governments, environments, cultures (particularly those related to food), and the creation of novel, safe, and efficient therapies that encourage weight loss and ameliorate the dysmetabolic state. These initiatives ought to be given top importance.

What Can You Do In This Regard?

There are techniques to increase the body's cells' receptivity to insulin, even if it may not be possible to completely overcome insulin resistance.

- The most effective strategy to fight insulin resistance is probably to get moving.

Long-term and short-term insulin resistance can both be significantly reduced by exercise. Physical activity increases the body's sensitivity to insulin, helps strengthen muscles that can absorb blood sugar, and creates a different pathway for glucose to enter muscle cells, reducing the need for insulin as a source of energy. Although this does not directly lower insulin resistance, it can aid those who already have it in controlling their blood sugar levels.

Additionally, losing weight also helps reduce insulin resistance. There is no diet that has been known to be the most efficient. Yet, other research indicates that consuming foods high in carbohydrates and low in fat may make insulin resistance worse. Moreover, studies have indicated that those who have weight-loss surgery are likely to develop much higher insulin sensitivity.

There are no drugs that are approved specifically to treat insulin resistance, although insulin sensitizers that are also diabetic drugs like metformin and thiazolidinediones, or TZDs, lower blood glucose levels by, at least in part, lowering insulin resistance.

- Never give up

Although it can be irritating and upsetting to battle an invisible opponent, realize that you are not alone. There are methods for overcoming insulin resistance. You can improve your health and blood glucose management by losing weight, getting more exercise, or using an insulin sensitizer.

- Alternate-day fasting

Intermittent fasting diets dramatically reduce insulin resistance and have specific therapeutic effects on blood glucose and lipids in patients with metabolic syndrome. It could be viewed as an adjunctive treatment for preventing the onset and progression of chronic illnesses.

- Eggs

They are a superior source of protein that contain all nine essential amino acids and have fewer than 0.5 grams of carbohydrates, making them perfect for shedding pounds and conquering insulin resistance.

CHAPTER 9

PREVENTING OBESITY

Due to gradual weight gain, a family history of obesity, a connected medical issue, or even simply a general concern for maintaining your health, you can be worried about preventing obesity. The aim is worthwhile regardless of your motivation. Reduce your risk of a variety of related health problems, including heart disease, diabetes, some cancers, and several other conditions, by preventing obesity.

Similar to many chronic illnesses, you can avoid obesity by leading a healthy lifestyle that includes regular exercise, nutritious food, obtaining enough sleep, and other factors. Whether you are already overweight or obese, the preventative and treatment measures remain the same.

The prevention of obesity is the subject of increasing amounts of research. According to the World Health Organization (WHO), the illness has spread globally and now affects more than 650 million people.

Diet

Obesity can be avoided by adhering to the fundamentals of good nutrition. These are some easy modifications you may make to your eating routine to aid in weight loss and the prevention of obesity.

- Concentrate on consuming five to seven servings of whole fruits and vegetables every day, or at least five. Foods that have fewer calories consist of fruits and vegetables. Consuming fruits and vegetables lowers the risk of obesity, according to the WHO. They have higher nutrient contents and are linked to a lower risk for diabetes and insulin resistance. They have more fiber than other foods, which makes you feel satisfied with fewer calories and helps you avoid gaining weight.

- Avoid processed foods:

Highly processed foods are a common source of empty calories, which tend to accumulate quickly. Examples include white bread and many boxed snack foods. According to a 2019 study, participants who were given a highly processed diet ate more calories and gained weight, whereas those who were given a minimally processed diet ate fewer calories and shed pounds.

- Limit your sugar intake

It is critical to limit your intake of added sugars. The American Heart Association advises against exceeding six teaspoons of added sugar per day for women and nine teaspoons per day for men. Other major sources of added sugar to stay away from are grain desserts like pies, cookies, and cakes, fruit drinks (which are rarely 100% fruit juice), candy, and dairy desserts like ice cream.

- Reduce your intake of artificial sweeteners because they have been associated with diabetes and obesity. If you must use a sweetener, choose a small amount of honey instead, which is a healthy substitute.
- Avoid saturated fats

They are linked to obesity, according to a 2018 study5. Instead, eat more monounsaturated and polyunsaturated fats from sources like avocados, olive oil, and tree nuts. Even good fats should only make up 20% to 35% of daily calories, and those who have vascular disease or high cholesterol may require even less.

- Drink wisely

Increase your water intake, and cut out any sugar-sweetened beverages from your diet. Make water your preferred beverage, decaffeinated tea and coffee are also acceptable. Avoid energy drinks and sports drinks since they not only have tons of added sugar but also, in the case of the former, have been linked to potential risks to the cardiovascular system.

- Prepare meals at home

Research on the frequency of meal preparation at home has shown that men and women who did so were less likely to acquire weight. They also had a lower risk of getting type 2 diabetes.

- Consider adopting a plant-based diet

Consuming a plant-based diet has been linked to better overall health and significantly lower obesity rates. Fill your plate with entire fruits and veggies at every meal to achieve this. Consume tiny amounts of unsalted nuts, such as almonds, cashews, walnuts, and pistachios—all of which are good for your heart—for snacks (1.5 ounces or a small handful). Red meat and dairy products, which are high in saturated fats, should be consumed in moderation (or not at all).

- Exercise

The majority of national and international guidelines suggest that the typical adult engages in 150 minutes or more of moderate-intensity exercise each week. Hence, five days a week, for at least 30 minutes per

day. According to research, brisk walking is the most effective exercise for keeping a healthy weight Studies discovered that those who walk quickly or briskly are more likely to be lighter, have a lower body mass index (BMI), and have smaller waists than people who engage in other types of exercise.
A standing desk, frequent stretch breaks, or finding ways to include walking meetings into your day are all further suggestions made by experts for staying active throughout the day.

- Relax

Cortisol levels rise as a result of ongoing stress, which also causes weight gain. Cortisol and other stress hormones can intensify "carb cravings" and make it challenging to use sound judgment and control, which can lead to bad eating decisions.

Look at the many healthy ways to reduce stress and determine which one suits you the most. Take daily walks, regularly practice yoga or tai chi, meditate, listen to your favorite music, spend time with friends, or do anything else that makes you feel calm and happy.

According to studies, owning a pet helps reduce blood pressure. Also, having a pet, particularly a dog, can boost your level of physical activity and prevent weight gain.

- Sleep

It is impossible to overestimate the importance of sleep for general health. This also applies to the purpose of preventing obesity. The Centers for Disease Control and Prevention advise adults over the age of 18 to get seven hours of sleep every night or more, and even more for children.

Research has connected later bedtimes to long-term weight increases. A later average bedtime during the workweek, measured in hours, from adolescence to adulthood was linked to an increase in BMI over time, according to one study that monitored over 3,500 teenagers between 1994 and 2009.

In another study, researchers discovered that children aged 4 and 5 who had later bedtimes experienced less sleep each night, which eventually increased their risk of becoming obese. In particular, the researchers discovered that children who slept less than 9.5 hours per night and kids who went to bed at 9 p.m. had higher odds of developing obesity later on in life.

- Reduce Screen Time

Although watching television (TV) can be entertaining and educational, it can also put your weight in danger It is an entirely sedentary activity that also seems to encourage unhealthy eating because of the frequent promotion of high-calorie, low-nutrient foods and beverages through advertisements, product placements, and other forms of advertising.

Use the following advice to reduce your child's exposure to TV and other screen media (including video games, leisure computer use, and similar activities)

All grownups: Limit your daily time spent watching television or using screens to two hours. The better, the less.

Parents:

No more than two hours should be spent watching screens by kids each day. The better, the less. Underage viewers should not watch any.

Make sure that kids' rooms are TV and Internet-free.

Do not watch TV while eating

Foods That Fight Obesity

Most of us actively try to restrict our intake of takeaways and snacks and are constantly looking for new strategies to burn fat. Knowing which foods to eat more of and which ones actively burn fat and calories is also beneficial.

- Fibre

When it comes to weight loss, fiber is king. It slows down digestion and prolongs the duration of your feeling satisfied. When decreasing calories, a frequent strategy for weight loss, which is highly significant.

- Chicory Seeds:

Two tablespoons of chia seeds, in one meal, deliver a whopping 40% of your daily fiber requirements. Together with delicacies like puddings, berry jams, and energy balls, it is very simple to include in meals, particularly breakfasts, and snacks.

- Fish:

Every week, we advise consuming two servings of seafood. Omega-3 fatty acids are found in fish like salmon, sardines, and tuna, and they not only improve heart and brain health but also aid in weight loss. Protein-rich foods like seafood can satisfy your appetite and keep you feeling full for a long time.

- Vegetables:

Brussels sprouts, broccoli and cauliflower greens with a dark color, such as kale and arugula, are examples of cruciferous vegetables. With a growing body of evidence demonstrating that regular eating of these veggies lowers the risk of cancer and reduces inflammation, their health advantages are immense. These vegetables are free of starch and aid in any weight loss program. Planning for these vegetables throughout the week is simple. Use as a robust base for salads that are meal-prepped, a low-carb alternative to grains, or blended into smoothies.

- Quinoa with grains:

Whole grains contain fiber that fills us up in addition to vitamins, minerals, and phytonutrients. Examples include whole-grain pasta, brown rice, and quinoa. Additionally, eating these foods alongside protein and healthy fats can help lessen cravings for refined carbs and sugar because our bodies and brains prefer the energy that carbohydrates provide.

- Apples:

Fruits can be a wise addition to a healthy weight loss diet, just like vegetables. Because they are inexpensive, can be stored for weeks in the refrigerator, and make a handy travel snack, apples are a particularly smart choice for a week's worth of meals. You might also think outside the box and include it in your diet.

Apples taste great in smoothies and salads. Apples are low in calories and low in filling because of their high water and fiber content (be sure to eat the skin).

- Pistachio:

Each type of nut can be a part of a balanced diet to help you lose weight. You feel satisfied because the food contains protein and fiber. As a serving of nuts (about one-fourth cup) contains between 160 and 200 calories, moderation is essential. Pistachios are one of the lowest-calorie nuts with 160 calories per serving. In addition to being delicious, pistachios provide many health advantages. According to studies, these unblemished green nuts may lower cholesterol levels, support a healthy gut, and help prevent type 2 diabetes.

Also, eating more than twice a week can lower your chance of gaining weight later on. Pistachios should be purchased whole since eating them while paying attention to your food is a mindful practice.

- Eggs

When it comes to weight loss, eggs are the ideal protein. It has been demonstrated that eating eggs for breakfast as part of a calorie-restricted diet helps people lose weight. Also, filling up high-protein breakfast items like eggs might help prevent nighttime snack cravings. It can be finished in a power bowl.

- Avocado:

It appears that avocado is a healthy complement to practically any diet. cause? They offer the benefits of both fiber and healthful fat, as well as a buttery texture that gives meals and snacks a richer flavor.

- Chocolate:

If a nutritious diet for weight loss can be maintained over the long term, it may be more effective. Any dietary or food group deficiency can cause intense desires, and continual abstinence from that food might result in binge eating. to support you in sticking to your weight loss goal. The indulgence you need to keep on track can be adding an ounce of dark chocolate. Also, you can benefit from heart health and mood-lifting.

The aforementioned foods must be included in your diet if you want to live a long and healthy life.

CONCLUSION

Making adjustments is a challenging task. Humans tend to reject change and avoid unfamiliar territory. You could have been shocked to find that other family members were not encouraging you if you have been attempting to alter your actions. Bear in mind that these unsupportive family members may be afraid of the changes you will need to make in order for them to love you when you succeed. A crucial first step in overcoming resistance to change and sabotage is communicating with your family about the reasons for the changes you are making.

When it comes to weight and health, family ties are very strong. A family affair, increasing nutrition through nutritious meals, organizing enjoyable and active activities, and supporting one another in your efforts! Decide on the first adjustment you will all make for better health today and take action!
Obesity has a genetic component, but this is just one of many risk factors. While some genes may influence a person's propensity to become obese, lifestyle variables still have a significant impact on obesity and can help mitigate hereditary risk factors.

Change the snack. Many people eat one or more snacks in between meals. As long as you select options that will fill you with fewer calories, snacking is acceptable. The trick is to eat healthy snacks. Opt for a (250 mg) cup of air-popped popcorn (31 calories), a cup (250 mg) of grapes and a low-fat cheese stick, or a small apple and 12 almonds in instead of a 3-ounce (85 g) bag of flavored tortilla chips (425 calories) (160 calories). You can easily save 500 calories a day by ingesting nutritious snacks twice a day.

Reduce one calorie-dense treat. Everyday, try to remove one food item with a lot of calories from your diet. Cutting off the donut in the morning, the brownie or bag of chips at lunch, or the chocolate cake at supper, will make you lose 250 to 350 calories. After lunch or dinner, go for a 40-minute brisk walk to burn an additional 150 calories.

Avoid drinking calories. A 16-ounce (475 mL) flavored latte can contain 250 calories or more, while a 12-ounce (355 mL) ordinary drink contains roughly 150 calories. Calories from drinking a few sugary drinks each day can quickly reach 500 or more. Save your calories for items that will make you feel full by substituting plain or flavored water, sparkling water, black coffee, or tea.
Use low-calorie alternatives. Switch some of your best high-calorie foods with lower-calorie alternatives. Use plain low-fat yogurt or Greek yogurt in place of, for instance, a cup (250 mL) of sour cream in a dish if it has a calorie count of 444. (154 calories).

Most restaurants serve quantities that are substantially bigger than what is advised. Ask the server to put half of your plate in a container so you may take it home and use it for another meal rather than finishing the entire food. A huge salad plus an appetiser can be used to form a dinner or you can split an entree with a companion. Just remember to use minimal amounts of dressing and fried garnishes.

Just avoid fried foods. Any dish that is fried contains a lot of unwanted calories and saturated fat. Choose grilled, broiled, or poached chicken or fish in place of fried. Likewise, omit the French fries. A meal's calories can increase by nearly 500 only from a hefty dish of fries. Instead, try to make do with a side salad or the vegetable of the day.

 Build the pizza thinner. Instead of deep-dish crust, more cheese, and meat toppings, go for a few pieces of vegetable-only thin-crust pizza. A bit more than 500 calories will be saved.
Eat all meals and snacks from a plate or bowl. It is simple to eat more than you intended to when you nibble from a bag or box. This usually occurs when you are watching TV whilst eating. The fact that a large bag of chips may contain more than 1000

calories may surprise you. Instead, put one serving in a bowl and the remainder in storage.

Skip the alcohol. Large number of people prefer cutting back on alcohol as a simple approach to losing weight. Alcohol has no nutritional value, so when you imbibe (drink) it, you are consuming empty calories. Most fruit drinks and juices made with syrup and sweeteners, ice cream, or heavy cream can have as many as 500 calories. Go for a 5-ounce (145 mL) glass of wine or a 12-ounce (355 mL) light beer (103 calories) (120 calories) anytime you want to order a drink
However, keep in mind that it is crucial to speak with a healthcare provider if you have made major lifestyle changes and are still gaining weight or struggling to lose weight. An underlying medical problem, such as an endocrine disorder or one that results in fluid retention, could be present.

Keep in mind that leading an active lifestyle is crucial for overall health, healthy weight management, and weight loss. For optimal outcomes, combine exercise with your weight loss attempts.